Vegan Cookbook For Beginners

*Easy And Delicious Vegan Recipes To Boost Your
Healthy*

Gwyneth Evans

© Copyright 2021 - All rights reserved.

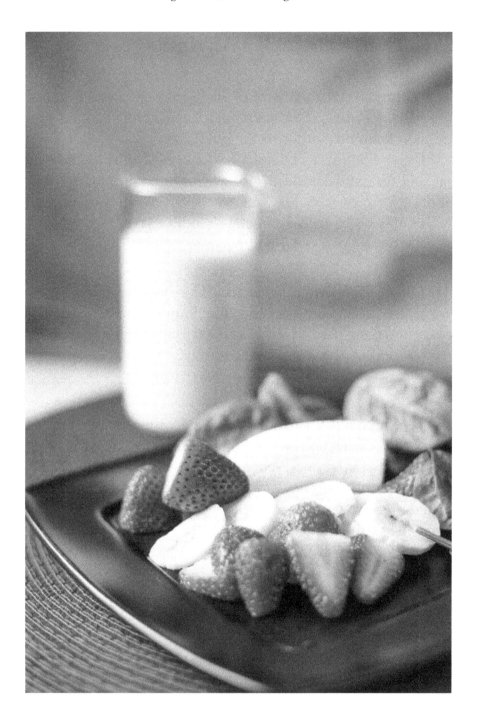

Table of Contents

Introduction

There are plenty of reasons why a vegan diet is worth following. First and foremost, eating vegan is good for our health. A vegan diet foregoes many high cholesterol and saturated fat that we would be eating on a standard diet. If we eat a well-rounded assortment of vegan foods, research has shown that we are more likely to have "lower blood pressure and cholesterol, and lower rates of heart disease, type 2 diabetes and some types of cancer" (The Vegan Society, n.d., para. 2). If you were previously eating an unhealthy diet before converting to veganism, you can also shed some extra pounds and get your beach body back!

We are also taking a stand against animal cruelty by using the power of our dollar. When we reject animal products at the grocery store and in restaurants, we tell the owners of these establishments that we don't support the animal cruelty inherent in the meat and dairy industry. We say no to factory farms that keep animals packed together in cages with a low quality of life. The vegan lifestyle is more ethical for animals and people alike.

In short, eating vegan isn't just good for us. It's good for the world around us. Just by eating vegan, we improve our health and the planet's health, making eating vegan all the more worthwhile.

Some people believe that eating vegan is confusing because there are many foods we don't eat. However, choosing vegan-compliant foods and ensuring all our meals are vegan is very simple. To eat vegan means eating a plant-based diet that doesn't include anything that came from an animal. Therefore, we only have to avoid two types of food: meat and animal products.

Avoiding meat is the easiest part of eating vegan, as it's very clear what is meat and what isn't. You can't eat chicken, beef, lamb, pork, venison, bison, or any other meat type. You also can't eat fish or shellfish. While this might initially seem to limit your choices at the grocery store, it encourages you to try different proteins you never considered before, expanding your palate and making mealtime more exciting. Many vegans find that after a few months of eating a meatless diet, their taste for meat disappears, and it no longer seems appetizing. This makes it incredibly easy to avoid, even if you were a devout carnivore before. Of course, avoiding meat isn't enough to make you a vegan—this would make you a vegetarian. Vegans take their diets one step further and also excise any animal products.

An animal product is anything produced by an animal. This includes dairy products made with cow or goat milk, chicken or duck eggs, fish eggs, honey from bees, and more. It also includes animal by-products that can be hidden in foods like rennet, gelatin, and isinglass, a chemical derived from fish bladders often present in beer. Though it is not technically part of your diet, many vegans also choose to forego non-food items made from animal products or through animal cruelty, such as makeup tested on animals, anything dyed red with carmine, and leather products.

Though there are quite a few foods you can't have as a vegan, you can also have hundreds of foods, so you can still make plenty of delicious meals. Instead of meat, you can eat tofu and other soy versions of meat products. Instead of honey, many vegans use agave or other sweeteners. It's very easy to eat vegan so long as you stick to the basic rules, and the lifestyle is far less restrictive than many similar diets.

CHAPTER 1:

Breakfast

1. Oatmeal Fruit Shake

Preparation Time: 10 minutes

Cooking Time: 0 minutes

Servings: 2

Ingredients:

- 1 cup oatmeal
- 1 apple, cored
- 1 banana, halved
- 1 cup baby spinach
- 2 cups coconut water
- 2 cups ice, cubed
- ½ tsp ground cinnamon
- 1 tsp pure vanilla extract

Directions

1. Blend all ingredients to a blender until smooth.

Nutrition:

270 Calories

1.5g Fats

5g Protein

2. Amaranth Banana Breakfast Porridge

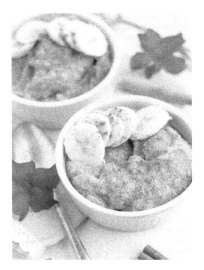

Preparation Time: 10 minutes

Cooking Time: 25 minutes

Servings: 8

Ingredients:

- 2 cup amaranth
- 2 cinnamon sticks
- 4 bananas, diced
- 2 Tbsp chopped pecans
- 4 cups water

Directions

1. Combine the amaranth, water, and cinnamon sticks, and banana in a pot. Cover and simmer around 25 minutes.

2. Remove from heat and discard the cinnamon. Places into bowls, and top with pecans.

Nutrition:

330 Calories

6g Fats

10g Protein

3. Breakfast Quinoa with Figs

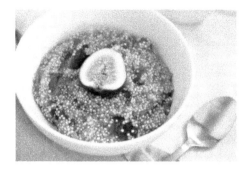

Preparation Time: 5 minutes

Cooking Time: 15 minutes

Servings: 4

Ingredients:

- 2 cups water
- 1 cup white quinoa
- 1 cup dried figs
- 1 cup walnuts
- 1 cup almond milk
- ½ tsp. cinnamon
- ¼ tsp. cloves

Directions

1. Rinse quinoa under cool water.
2. Combine it with water, cinnamon, and cloves. Bring to boil.
3. Simmer covered for 10-15 minutes.

4. Add dried figs, nuts, and milk.

Nutrition:

420 Calories

20g Fats

11g Protein

4. Spiced Quinoa Porridg

Preparation Time: 30 minutes Cooking Time: 30 minutes Servings:4 Ingredients:

- ¾ cup uncooked quinoa
- 1/8 teaspoon ground cardamom
- 1½ cups water
- ½ teaspoon ground cinnamon
- ¼ teaspoon ground ginger
- 1/8 teaspoon ground cloves
- 2 tablespoon ground sunflower seeds
- 2 tablespoons maple syrup
- ¼ cup fresh strawberries, hulled and sliced

Directions

1. Put water, quinoa and spices in a medium pan over medium heat.
2. Bring to a boil and reduce the heat to low.
3. Simmer, for 20 minutes and remove from the heat.
4. Stir in the sunflower seeds, maple syrup and strawberries to serve.

Nutrition: 169 Calories 15.4g Fat 7.5g Protein

5. Fruit Cup

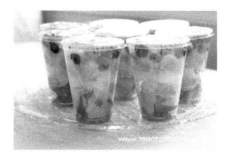

Preparation Time: 15 Minutes Cooking Time: 0 minute

Servings: 4   Ingredients:

- 2 cups melon
- 2 cups strawberries
- 2 cups grapes, sliced in half
- 2 cups peaches, sliced
- 3 tablespoons lime juice
- ½ teaspoon ground ginger
- 3 teaspoons lime zest
- ¼ cup coconut flakes, toasted

Directions

1. Toss the fruits in lime juice, ginger.
2. Sprinkle the lime zest on top.
3. Top with the coconut flakes.

Nutrition:

65 Calories 1.6g Fiber 1g Protein

6. Simple Vegan Breakfast Hash

Preparation Time: 10 minutes

Cooking Time: 25 minutes

Servings: 4

Ingredients:

For Potatoes:

- 1 large sweet potato
- 3 medium potatoes
- 1 tablespoon onion powder
- 2 teaspoons sea salt
- 1 tablespoon garlic powder
- 1 teaspoon ground black pepper
- 1 teaspoon dried thyme
- 1/4 cup olive oil

For Skillet Mixture:

- 1 medium onion
- 5 cloves of garlic
- ¼ teaspoon salt
- ¼ teaspoon black pepper
- 1 teaspoon olive oil

Directions:

1. Switch on the oven, then set it to 450 degrees F and let it preheat.
2. Meanwhile, take a casserole dish, add all the ingredients for the potatoes, toss, and then cook for 20 minutes, stirring halfway.
3. Meanwhile, take a skillet pan, place it over medium heat, add oil and when hot, cook onion and garlic, for 5 minutes, season well.
4. When potatoes have roasted, add garlic and cooked onion mixture, stir, and serve.

Nutrition:

212 Calories

10g Fat

3g Protein

7. Peanut Butter Granola

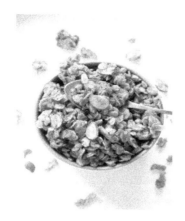

Preparation Time: 10 Minutes

Cooking Time: 47 minutes

Servings: 4

Ingredients:

- 4 cups oats
- 1/3 cup of cocoa powder
- ¾ cup peanut butter
- 1/3 cup maple syrup
- 1/3 cup avocado oil
- 1½ teaspoons vanilla extract
- ½ cup cocoa nibs
- 6 ounces dark chocolate

Directions

1. Preheat your oven to 300 degrees F.

2. Spray a baking sheet with cooking spray.

3. In a medium saucepan add oil, maple syrup, and peanut butter.

4. Cook for 2 minutes on medium heat, stirring.

5. Add the oats and cocoa powder, mix well.

6. Spread the coated oats on the baking sheet.

7. Bake for 45 minutes, occasionally stirring.

8. Garnish with dark chocolate, cocoa nibs, and peanut butter.

Nutrition:

134 Calories

4.7g Fat 6.2g Protein

8. Apple Chia Pudding

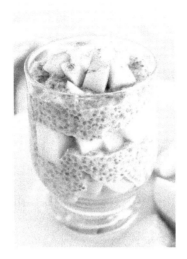

Preparation Time: 10 minutes

Cooking Time: 5 minutes

Servings: 4

Ingredients:

Chia Pudding:

- 4 tablespoons chia seeds

- 1 cup almond milk

- ½ teaspoon cinnamon

- Apple Filling:

- 1 large apple

- ¼ cup water

- 2 teaspoons maple syrup

- Pinch cinnamon
- 2 tablespoons golden raisins

Directions

1. In a sealable container, add cinnamon, chia seeds and almond milk, mix well.
2. Seal the container and refrigerate overnight.
3. In a medium pot, combine all apple pie filling ingredients and cook for 5 minutes.
4. Serve the chia pudding with apple filling on top.

Nutrition:

387 Calories

2.9g Fiber

6.6g Protein

9. Pumpkin Spice Bites

Preparation Time: 10 minutes

 Cooking Time: 0 minutes

Servings: 2

Ingredients:

- ½ cup pumpkin puree

- ½ cup almond butter

- ¼ cup maple syrup

- 1 teaspoon pumpkin pie spice

- 1 1/3cup rolled oats

- 1/3 cup pumpkin seeds

- 1/3 cup raisins

- 2 tablespoons chia seeds

Directions

1. In a sealable container, add everything and mix well.

2. Seal the container and refrigerate overnight.

3. Roll the mixture into small balls.

4. Serve.

Nutrition: 212 Calories 4.4g Fibers 7.3g Protein

10.No-Bake Vegan Protein Bar

Preparation Time: 20 minutes

Cooking Time: 0 minute

Serving: 5

Ingredients:

- 1/3 cup amaranth

- 3 tbsp. vanilla vegan protein powder.

- 2 tbsp maple syrup.

- 1 cup almond butter.

- 3 tbsp. dark vegan chocolate.

Direction:

1. In 8 x 8-inch baking pan, place parchment paper and set aside.

2. Pop your amaranth by heating a big pot over medium-high heat.

3. Include about 2-3 tbsp amaranth at a time and right away cover. Shake over the heat to move the grain around.

4. Not every single grain will pop.

5. Do not blend any scorched grain with the completely popped grain. Set aside.

6. Mix in almond butter and maple syrup. Then add protein powder and stir.

7. Include popped amaranth a little at a time until you have a loose "dough" texture.

8. Transfer the mixture to the baking meal and press down to form an even layer. Lay parchment paper or plastic wrap on the top.

9. Transfer to freezer to set for 10-15 minutes or until firm to the touch. Lift out and slice it into nine bars.

Nutrition:

215 Calories

15g Fat

10.7g Protein

11. Orange Pumpkin Pancakes

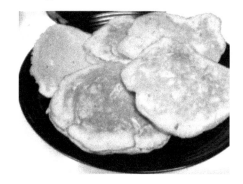

Preparation Time: 15 minutes

Cooking Time: 10 minutes

Serving: 4

Ingredients:

- 10 g ground flax meal

- 45 ml water

- 235 ml unsweetened soy milk

- 15 ml lemon juice

- 60 g buckwheat flour

- 60 g all-purpose flour

- 8 g baking powder

- 2 tsp finely grated orange zest

- 25 g white chia seeds

- 120 g organic pumpkin puree

- 30 ml melted and cooled coconut oil

- 5 ml vanilla paste
- 30 ml pure maple syrup

Direction

1. Combine ground flax meal with water. Place aside for 10 minutes. Combine almond milk and cider vinegar. Place aside for 5 minutes.
2. Mix buckwheat flour, all-purpose flour, baking powder, orange zest, and chia seeds.
3. Whisk almond milk, along with pumpkin puree, coconut oil, vanilla, and maple syrup.
4. Heat large non-stick skillet over medium-high heat. Brush the skillet gently with some coconut oil.
5. Pour 60ml of batter into skillet. Cook the pancake for 1 minute. Flip.
6. Cook 1 1/2 minutes more. Slide the pancake onto a plate. Repeat with the remaining batter.

Nutrition:

301 Calories

12.6g fat

8.1g Protein

12. Sweet Potato Slices with Fruits

Preparation Time: 15 minutes

Cooking Time: 10 minutes

Serving: 2

Ingredients:

- 1 sweet potato

Topping.

- 60 g organic peanut butter.
- 30ml pure maple syrup.
- 4 dried apricots, sliced.
- 30 g fresh raspberries

Direction

1. Peel and slice sweet potato into 1/2 cm thick slices.
2. Place the potato slices in a toaster on high for 5 minutes. Toast your sweet potatoes TWICE.
3. Arrange sweet potato slices onto a plate.
4. Spread the peanut butter over sweet potato slices.
5. Drizzle the maple syrup over the butter. Top each slice with an equal amount of sliced apricots and raspberries. Serve.

Nutrition: 300 Calories 16.9g fat 10.3g Protein

13.Energizing Daily Tonic

Preparation Time: 15 minutes

Cooking Time: 0 minute

Serving: 2

Ingredients base:

- 2-4 tbsp. vegan protein powder.

- 1 tbsp. maca powder.

- 1 tsp. ashwagandha powder.

- 1 tsp. mushroom blend powder.

- 1 tsp. astragalus powder.

- 1/4 cup pecans.

- 2 Brazil nuts.

- Pinch of stevia powder.

- 1-2 tbsp. maple syrup or dates

Add-ons:

- 1 tbsp. cacao powder.

- 1 tbsp. ground coffee.

- 1/2 tsp. vanilla extract.

Direction

1. Blend all the base active ingredients except the maple syrup up until smooth, velvety and tasty. Include 1 to 2 tablespoons of maple syrup or a small handful of dates, if you desire it sweeter.

2. Sprinkle with apple pie spice, if utilizing, and enjoy!

Nutrition

160 Calories

5.5g Protein

0.8g fat

14.Strawberry Maple Scones

Preparation Time: 10 minutes

Cooking Time: 15 minutes

Serving: 6

Ingredients:

- 2 cups oat flour.

- 1/3 cup almond milk.

- 1 cup of strawberries.

- A handful of dried currants.

- 5 tbsp. coconut oil.

- 5 tbsp. of maple syrup.

- 1 tbsp. baking powder.

- 1 1/2 tsp. vanilla extract.

- 1 tsp. cinnamon.

Direction

1. Include the coconut oil and with a pastry cutter or fork, cut and blend the coconut oil into the oat flour mix until a crumbly dough form. Mix in strawberry pieces, currants and slowly include in all the wet ingredients. Slowly blend the dry and wet components.

2. On a prepared baking sheet with parchment paper, form a circle out of the dough - it must have to do with 1 inch thick. Cut into eight triangular pieces and bake for 15-17 minutes. Delight in with jam, nut butter!

Nutrition:

342 Calories

48g Carbohydrates

4.1g Protein

15.Spinach Tofu Scramble with Sour Cream

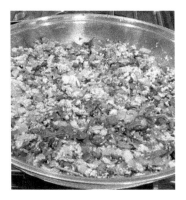

Preparation Time: 10 minutes Cooking Time: 20 minutes

Serving: 4

Sour cream:

- 75 g raw cashews

- 30 ml lemon juice

- 5 g nutritional yeast

- 60 ml water 1 pinch salt

Tofu scramble:

- 15 ml olive oil.

- 1 small onion

- 1 clove garlic.

- 400 firm tofu

- 1/2 tsp. ground cumin.

- 1/2 tsp. curry powder.

- 1/2 tsp. turmeric.
- 2 tomatoes, diced.
- 30 g baby spinach

Direction

1. Make the cashew sour cream; rinse and drain soaked cashews.
2. Place the cashews, lemon juice, nutritional yeast, water, and salt in a food processor.
3. Blend on high until smooth, for 5-6 minutes.
4. Transfer to a bowl and place aside. Make the tofu scramble; heat olive oil in a skillet.
5. Add onion and cook 5 minutes over medium-high.
6. Add garlic, and cook stirring, for 1 minute.
7. Stir in crumbled tofu to coat with oil.
8. Add the cumin, curry, and turmeric. Cook the tofu for 2 minutes.
9. Cook tomatoes for 2 minutes.
10. Add spinach and cook, tossing until completely wilted, about 1 minute. Transfer tofu scramble on the plate. Top with a sour cream and serve.

Nutrition:

411 Calories 26g fat 25g Protein

CHAPTER 2:

Lunch

16.Mushroom Cream

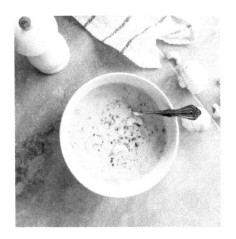

Preparation Time: 10 minutes

Cooking Time: 20 minutes

Serving: 2

Ingredients

- 2 teaspoons olive oil

- 1 onion

- 2 garlic cloves

- 2 cups chopped mushrooms

- 2 tablespoons whole-grain flour
- 1 teaspoon dried herbs
- 4 cups Economical Vegetable Broth
- 1½ cups nondairy milk

Direction

1. Preheat oil over medium-high heat.
2. Add the onion, garlic, mushrooms, and salt. Sauté for about 5 minutes, until softened. Throw flour over the ingredients in the pot and mix.
3. Cook for 1 to 2 minutes more to toast the flour.
4. Add the dried herbs, vegetable broth, milk, and pepper.
5. Set heat to low, and let the broth come to a simmer.
6. Cook for 10 minutes, until slightly thickened.

Nutrition:

127 Calories

10g Protein

3g Fiber

17.Fast Twitch Quinoa

Preparation Time: 5 minutes

Cooking Time: 0 minute

Serving: 7

Ingredients

- 3 tablespoons olive oil
- Juice of 1½ lemons
- 1 teaspoon garlic powder
- ½ teaspoon dried oregano
- 1 bunch curly kale
- 2 cups cooked tricolor quinoa
- 1 cup canned mandarin oranges in juice
- 1 cup diced yellow summer squash
- 1 red bell pepper
- ½ red onion
- ½ cup dried cranberries
- ½ cup slivered almonds

Direction

1. Scourge the oil, lemon juice, garlic powder, and oregano.

2. Mix the kale with the oil-lemon mixture until well coated. Add the quinoa, oranges, squash, bell pepper, and red onion and toss until all the ingredients are well combined. Divide among bowls or transfer to a large serving platter. Top with the cranberries and almonds.

Nutrition:

343 Calories

24g Protein

11g Fiber

18.Eggplant Parmesan

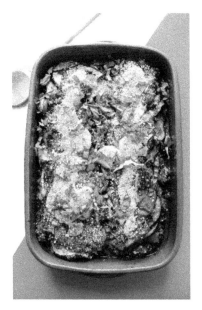

Preparation Time: 10 minutes

Cooking Time: 15 minutes Serving: 1

Ingredients

- ¼ cup nondairy milk

- ¼ cup bread crumbs or panko

- 2 tablespoons nutritional yeast

- ¼ teaspoon salt

- 4 (¼-inch-thick) eggplant slices

- 1 tablespoon olive oil

- 4 tablespoons Simple Homemade Tomato Sauce

- 4 teaspoons Pram Sprinkle

Direction

1. Put the milk in a shallow bowl. Blend the bread crumbs, nutritional yeast and salt.

2. Dip one eggplant slice in the milk, making sure both sides get moistened. Dip it into the bread crumbs, flipping to coat both sides. Transfer to a plate and repeat to coat the remaining slices. Pre-heat oil over medium heat and add the breaded eggplant slices.

3. Cook for 6 minutes. Flip, adding more oil as needed. Top each slice with 1 tablespoon tomato sauce and 1 teaspoon Pram Sprinkle.

4. Cook for 5 to 7 minutes more.

Nutrition:

460 Calories

9g Protein

13g Fiber

19.Pepper & Kale

Preparation Time: 5 minutes

Cooking Time: 15 minutes

Serving: 4

Ingredients

- 2 cans chickpeas

- 4 cloves garlic

- 1 large sweet onion

- 4 tbsp olive oil

- 2 red peppers

- 6 cups kale

Direction

1. Heat BBQ and prepare a greased BBQ basket or pan.

2. Meanwhile, mix together chickpeas, garlic, onion, red peppers and olive oil in a bowl and add to the BBQ basket and place on the grill. Stir regularly.

3. When almost ready to serve add kale and stir constantly until the kale is slightly wilted. Serve with garlic toast, pita bread or rice.

Nutrition: 520 Calories 16g Fiber 18g Protein

20.   Caesar Pasta

Preparation Time: 10 minutes

Cooking Time: 0 minute

Serving: 1

Ingredients

- 2 cups chopped romaine lettuce
- 2 tablespoons Vegan Caesar Dressing
- ½ cup cooked pasta
- ½ cup canned chickpeas
- 2 additional tablespoons Caesar Dressing

Direction

1. Blend the lettuce, dressing, (if using).
2. Add the pasta, chickpeas, and additional dressing. Toss to coat.

Nutrition:

415 Calories

9g Protein

13g Fiber

21. Quinn-Otto with Dried Tomatoe

Preparation Time: 10 minutes

Cooking Time: 30 min

Serving: 2

Ingredients

- 3 cups vegetable broth

- 2 cloves garlic, minced

- ½ cup quinoa

- ¼ cup sun-dried tomatoes in oil

- 1 teaspoon parsley

- 1 small onion, minced

- 1 ½ tablespoons olive oil

- 2 tablespoons basil

Direction

1. Place a saucepan over medium heat. Add oil. Once heated, sauté onion and garlic.

2. Cook the quinoa: Cook 2/3 cup uncooked quinoa in water, according to package directions.

3. Add a cup of broth and mix well. Season.

4. Add some more broth, tomatoes and herbs. Mix well. Cook until nearly dry.

5. Repeat adding the broth, a little at a time and cook until nearly dry each time, add cooked quinoa. Stir often.

Nutrition:

402 Calories

13g Fat

11g Protein

22.   Steamed Eggplants with Peanut Dressing

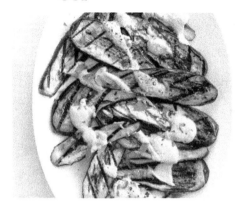

Preparation Time: 10 minutes

Cooking Time: 20 minutes

Serving: 2

Ingredients:

- 6 ounces baby eggplants
- ½ tablespoon soy sauce
- ½ teaspoon sugar
- 1 teaspoon toasted sesame seeds
- 1 tablespoon cilantro leaves, to garnish
- 1 tablespoon peanut butter
- ½ tablespoon rice vinegar
- ½ tablespoon chili oil + extra to serve
- 1 spring onion, thinly sliced
- 1 tablespoon boiling water

Direction

1. Steam the eggplants in the steaming equipment you possess for about 15 minutes or until soft.

2. Place peanut butter in a bowl. Add boiling water into it and whisk well.

3. Add soy sauce, sugar, rice vinegar and chili oil and whisk well.

4. Place the eggplants on a serving platter. Trickle the sauce mixture over the eggplants.

5. Sprinkle sesame seeds, cilantro, spring onion on top. Drizzle some chili oil on top and serve.

Nutrition:

87 Calories

3.8g Protein

2.9g Fiber

23. Cauliflower Rice Wok

Preparation Time: 10 minutes

Cooking Time: 20 minutes

Serving: 4

Ingredients

- 1 lb. (450 g) tofu
- 1/2 cup (150 g) peas
- 1 tablespoon ginger
- 3 garlic cloves, minced
- 1/4 cup (30 g) green onions
- 1 cauliflower head, riced
- 2 carrots, diced
- 2 tablespoons sesame oil
- 3 tablespoons cashews
- 3 tablespoons soy sauce

Direction

1. Press and drain the tofu. Then crumble it slightly in a bowl. Set aside.

2. Add oil to a wok pan and place over medium heat. Cook garlic and ginger. Add the tofu and stir for

about 6 minutes, until golden and well cooked. Set the tofu aside.

3. Fill more oil to the pan and cook the carrots.

4. Mix peas along with the cauliflower rice. Cook for 7 minutes. Add the green onions, cooked tofu, cashews and soy sauce.

5. Serve the cauliflower fried rice and garnish with the sesame seeds. Enjoy!

Nutrition:

47 Calories

2.14g Protein

3.2g Fiber

24. Spicy Root and Lentil Casserole

Preparation Time: 10 minutes

Cooking Time: 35 minutes

Serving: 4

Ingredients:

- 2 tbsp vegetable oil
- 1 onion, chopped
- 2 garlic cloves, crushed
- 700g potatoes, peeled and cut into chunks
- 4 carrot, thickly sliced
- 2 parsnip, thickly sliced
- 2 tbsp curry paste or powder
- 1 liter/1¾ pints vegetable stock
- 100g red lentils

Direction

1. Cook oil in a large pan, cook the onion and garlic over a medium heat for 3 minutes. Continue stirring in between to cook them well. Add potatoes, carrots and parsnips, turn up the heat and cook for 6 to 7 minutes. Stir well

2. Stir in the curry paste or powder, fill in the stock, and bring to a boil. Reduce the heat, add the lentils. Cover and simmer for 18 minutes.

3. Once done, season with coriander and heat for a minute. Serve with yogurt and the rest of the coriander.

Nutrition:

378 Calories

14g Protein

10g Fiber

25. Seitan

Preparation Time: 25 minutes

Cooking Time: 20 minutes

Serving: 5

Ingredients

- Firm Tofu, 250 grams

- Unsweetened soy milk, 150ml

- Miso paste 2 tsp

- Marmite 2 tsp

- Onion powder 1 tsp

- Garlic powder 2 tsp

- Wheat gluten 160g

- Pea protein or vegan protein powder, 40g

- Vegetable stock 1 ½ liters

Direction

1. Blitz the tofu, soy milk, miso, marmite, onion powder, garlic powder, 1 tsp salt and ½ tsp white pepper in a food processor. Blend until smooth.

2. Mix them all to form a dough. Knead the dough well, stretching and tearing for 10-15 minutes.

3. Fill vegetable stock into a pan and let it simmer. Flatten out the seitan to a thickness of 1 cm and

chop into chunks. Simmer it in the stock for 20 minutes covering with a lid. Once it's done, allow it to cool down. Chop or tear it into smaller pieces before cooking as per your choice.

Nutrition:

211Calories

35g Protein

2g Fiber

26. Gear Up Lentils

Preparation Time: 5 minutes Cooking Time: 40 minutes

Serving: 6

Ingredients

- 5 cups water
- 2¼ cups brown lentils
- 3 teaspoons minced garlic
- 1 bay leaf
- ½ teaspoon dried basil
- ½ teaspoon dried oregano
- ½ teaspoon dried rosemary
- ½ teaspoon dried thyme

Direction:

1. Boil water, lentils, garlic, bay leaf, basil, oregano, rosemary, and thyme. Decrease heat to low, and simmer for 35 minutes. Drain any excess cooking liquid.

2. Transfer to a container, or scoop 1 cup of lentils into each of 6 storage containers. Let cool before sealing the lids.

Nutrition: 257 Calories 1g Fat 19g Protein

27.   Boulders Bean Burgers

Preparation Time: 10 minutes

Cooking Time: 10 minutes Serving: 4

Ingredients

- 1 tablespoon olive oil
- ¼ cup couscous
- ¼ cup boiling water
- 1 (15-ounce) can white beans
- 2 tablespoons balsamic vinegar
- 2 tablespoons chopped sun-dried tomatoes or olives
- ½ teaspoon garlic powder
- ½ teaspoon salt
- 4 burger buns

Direction

1. Preheat the oven to 350°F.
2. Grease rimmed baking sheet with olive oil or line it with parchment paper. Mix couscous and boiling water.
3. Cover and set aside for about 5 minutes. Once the couscous is soft and the water is absorbed, fluff it with a fork. Add the beans, and mash them to a

chunky texture. Add the vinegar, olive oil, sun-dried tomatoes, garlic powder, and salt; stir until combined but still a bit chunky.

4. Portion mixture into 4, and shape each into a patty. Put the patties on the prepared baking sheet, and bake for 25 to 30 minutes. Alternatively, heat some olive oil in a large skillet over medium heat, then add the patties, making sure each has oil under it.

5. Fry for about 5 minutes. Flip, adding more oil as needed, and fry for about 5 minutes more. Serve.

Nutrition:

315 Calories 12g Fiber 16g Protein

28. Black Bean Pizza Plate

Preparation Time: 10 minutes

Cooking Time: 20 minutes Serving: 2

Ingredients

- 2 prebaked pizza crusts
- ½ cup Spicy Black Bean Dip
- 1 tomato, thinly sliced
- 1 carrot, grated
- 1 red onion
- 1 avocado

Direction

1. Preheat the oven to 400°F.
2. Lay the two crusts out on a large baking sheet. Spread half the Spicy Black Bean
3. Dip on each pizza crust.
4. Then layer on the tomato slices with a pinch pepper if you like. Sprinkle the grated carrot with the sea salt and lightly massage it in with your hands.
5. Spread the carrot on top of the tomato, then add the onion.
6. Pop the pizzas in the oven for 10 to 20 minutes, or until they're done to your taste.

7. Top the cooked pizzas with sliced avocado and another sprinkle of pepper.

Nutrition

379 Calories

15g Fiber

13g Protein

29.   Instant Peas Risotto

Preparation Time: 10 min.

Cooking Time: 10 min.

Servings: **3**

Ingredients:

- 1 cup baby green peas
- 1 cup Arborio rice
- 2 cloves garlic, diced
- 3 tablespoons olive oil
- 1 brown onion, diced
- ½ teaspoon salt
- 2 celery sticks, make small cubes
- ½ teaspoon pepper
- 2 tablespoons lemon juice
- **2 cups vegetable stock**

Directions:

1. Take your Instant Pot and place it on a clean kitchen platform. Turn it on after plugging it into a power socket.

2. Put the pot on "Saute" mode. In the pot, add the oil, celery, onions, pepper, and salt; cook for 4-5 minutes until the ingredients become soft.

3. Mix in the zest, stock, garlic, peas, and rice. Stir the ingredients.

4. Close the lid and lock. Ensure that you have sealed the valve to avoid leakage.

5. Press "Manual" mode and set timer for 5 minutes. It will take a few minutes for the pot to build inside pressure and start cooking.

6. After the timer reads zero, press "Cancel" and quick release pressure.

7. **Carefully remove the lid, add the lemon juice and serve warm!**

Nutrition:

Calories - 362

Fat – 13g

Carbohydrates – 52.5g

Fiber – 3g

Protein – 8g

30.   Pumpkin Bean Stew

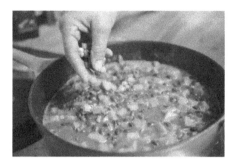

Preparation Time: 8-10 min.

Cooking Time: 20-22 min.

Servings: **4**

Ingredients:

- 2 cloves garlic, minced
- 3 cups water
- 2 medium tomatoes, chopped
- 1/2 cup dried chickpeas (soaked for 12 hours and drained)
- 3 small onions, chopped
- 1 cup raw pumpkin, peeled, cubed
- 1/2 cup dried navy beans (soaked for 12 hours and drained)
- Pepper and salt as needed
- 2 teaspoon harissa
- 2 tablespoons parsley, chopped

Directions:

1. Take your Instant Pot and place it on a clean kitchen platform. Turn it on after plugging it into a power socket. Put the pot on "Saute" mode. In the pot, add the oil, garlic, and onions; cook for 2-3 minutes until the ingredients become soft. Add other ingredients to the pot. Stir gently.

2. Close the lid and lock. Ensure that you have sealed the valve to avoid leakage.

3. Press "Bean/Chili" mode and set the timer for 6 minutes. It will take a few minutes for the pot to build inside pressure and start cooking.

4. After the timer reads zero, press "Cancel" and naturally release pressure. It takes about 8-10 minutes to naturally release pressure.

5. Carefully remove the lid.

6. Check if the beans are tender, if not add some more water; cook on "Manual" mode for 8-10 minutes.

7. Top with parsley and serve.

Nutrition: Calories - 166 Fat – 8g Carbohydrates – 24g Fiber – 6.5g Protein – 9g

CHAPTER 3:

Dinner

31.Spicy Black-Eyed Peas

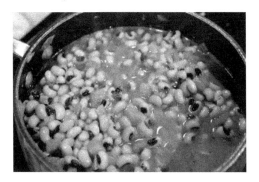

Preparation Time: 15 Minutes

Cooking Time: 60 Minutes

Servings: 8

Ingredients:

- 32-ounce black-eyed peas, uncooked

- 1 cup of chopped orange bell pepper

- 1 cup of chopped celery

- 8-ounce of chipotle peppers, chopped

- 1 cup of chopped carrot

- 1 cup of chopped white onion
- 1 teaspoon of minced garlic
- 3/4 teaspoon of salt
- 1/2 teaspoon of ground black pepper
- 2 teaspoons of liquid smoke flavoring
- 2 teaspoons of ground cumin
- 1 tablespoon of adobo sauce
- 2 tablespoons of olive oil
- 1 tablespoon of apple cider vinegar
- 4 cups of vegetable broth

Directions:

1. Place a medium-sized non-stick skillet pan over an average temperature of heat; add the bell peppers, carrot, onion, garlic, oil and vinegar.
2. Stir until it mixes properly and let it cook for 5 to 8 minutes or until it gets translucent.
3. Transfer this mixture to a 6-quarts slow cooker and add the peas, chipotle pepper, adobo sauce and the vegetable broth.
4. Stir until mixes properly and cover the top.

5. Plug in the slow cooker; adjust the cooking time to 8 hours and let it cook on the low heat setting or until peas are soft.

Nutrition:

Calories: 211

Carbs: 22g

Fat: 7g

Protein: 19g

32. Creamy Artichoke Soup

Preparation time: 5 minutes

Cooking time: 40 minutes

Servings: 4

Ingredients:

- 1 can artichoke hearts, drained
- 3 cups vegetable broth
- 2 tablespoon lemon juice
- 1 small onion, finely cut
- 2 cloves garlic, crushed
- 3 tablespoons olive oil
- 2 tablespoon flour
- 1/2 cup vegan cream

Directions:

1. Gently sauté the onion and garlic in some olive oil.

2. Add the flour, whisking constantly, and then add the hot vegetable broth slowly, while still whisking. Cook for about 5 minutes.

3. Blend the artichoke, lemon juice, salt and pepper until smooth. Add the puree to the broth mix, stir well, and then stir in the cream.

4. Cook until heated through. Garnish with a swirl of vegan cream or a sliver of artichoke.

Nutrition:

Calories: 211

Carbs: 12g

Fat: 7g

Protein: 11g

33. Super Rad-ish Avocado Salad

Preparation time: 10 minutes

Cooking time: 25 minutes

Servings: 2 Salads.

Ingredients:

- 6 shredded carrots

- 6 ounces diced radishes

- 1 diced avocado

- 1/3 cup ponzu

Directions:

1. Bring all the above **Ingredients:** together in a serving bowl and toss. Enjoy!

Nutrition:

Calories: 211

Carbs: 9g

Fat: 7g

Protein: 12g

34. Beauty School Ginger Cucumbers

Preparation time: 10 minutes

Cooking time: 5 minutes

Servings: 14 slices.

Ingredients:

- 1 sliced cucumber
- 3 teaspoon rice wine vinegar
- 1 1/2 tablespoon sugar
- 1 teaspoon minced ginger

Directions:

1. Bring all of the above **Ingredients:** together in a mixing bowl, and toss the **Ingredients:** well. Enjoy!

Nutrition:

Calories: 210

Carbs: 14g

Fat: 7g

Protein: 19g

35.   Mushroom Salad

Preparation time: 10 minutes

Cooking time: 20 minutes

Servings: 2

Ingredients:

- 1 tablespoon butter
- 1/2 pound cremini mushrooms, chopped
- 2 tablespoons extra-virgin olive oil
- Salt and black pepper to taste
- 2 bunches arugula
- 4 slices prosciutto
- 1 tablespoon apple cider vinegar
- 4 sundried tomatoes in oil, drained and chopped
- Fresh parsley leaves, chopped

Directions:

1. Heat a pan with butter and half of the oil.
2. Add the mushrooms, salt, and pepper. Stir-fry for 3 minutes. Reduce heat. Stir again, and cook for 3 minutes more.
3. Add rest of the oil and vinegar. Stir and cook for 1 minute.

4. Place arugula on a platter, add prosciutto on top, add the mushroom mixture, sundried tomatoes, more salt and pepper, parsley, and serve.

Nutrition:

Calories: 191

Carbs: 6g

Fat: 7g

Protein: 17g

CHAPTER 4:

Snacks

36.   Trail Mix

Preparation Time: 5 minutes

Cooking Time: 0 minute

Servings: 4

Ingredients

¼ cup of almonds

- ¼ cup of cashews

- ¼ cup of dried apricots

- ¼ cup of dried cranberries

- ¼ cup of pitted dates

Direction

1.Combine the almonds, cashews, cranberries, apricots, and dates in a bowl.

Nutrition

130 Calories 14.2g Carbohydrates

3.4g Protein

37. Veggie Crisps

Preparation Time: 5 minutes

Cooking Time: 20 minutes

Servings: 4

Ingredients:

- 2 medium carrots
- 1 medium beetroot
- 1 medium baby marrow
- 1 small sweet potato
- 1 small turnip
- 1-2 tsp of olive oil
- ½ tsp of black pepper
- ½ tsp of Himalayan salt

Direction

1.Preheat the oven to 350-400 degrees-Fahrenheit. In a baking tray, lay out parchment paper.

2.Slice the vegetables each into 1-inch slices with a sharp knife, and place them in a bowl.

3.Mix in olive oil and season the vegetables, coat well.

4.Arrange vegetables onto the baking sheet, and bake them for 10 minutes on one side. Then, turn over, and bake them for 6-8 minutes.

5.Remove the vegetable crisps from the oven, and allow them to cool down.

Nutrition

78 Calories 34g Carbohydrates

2.4g Protein

38. Tamari Almonds

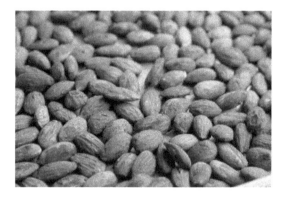

Preparation Time: 5 minutes   Cooking Time: 20 minutes

Servings: 4

Ingredients

- 400g of raw almonds

- ¼ cup of tamari sauce

- ¼ tsp of sea salt

Direction

1.Heat the oven to 180 degrees-Fahrenheit, and line a baking tray with parchment paper.   .Spread the almonds onto the baking tray, drizzle the tamari sauce over the nuts, and add the sea salt.   .Bake the almonds in the oven for 25 minutes, moving them around every 5 to 10 minutes until the tamari sauce is absorbed by the nuts. **Nutrition 115 Calories** 2.1g Carbohydrates 4.4g Protein

39. Sweet Tiffin

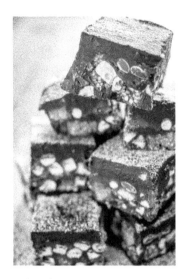

Preparation Time: 15 minutes

Cooking Time: 2 hours

Servings: 4

Ingredients

- 1 cup of dark chocolate (vegan)
- 2/3 cups of macadamia nuts
- 1/3 cup of dried cranberries
- 1/3 cup of coconut oil
- ¼ cup of pistachios
- 2 tbsp of maple syrup

Direction

1.Spray a brownie tin with cooking spray. Layer the tin with a single sheet of parchment paper.

2.Add the chocolate and maple syrup to a microwaveable bowl, and microwave it for 30 seconds or until you reach a smooth consistency.

3.Crush the nuts into smaller pieces in a bowl. Add the cranberries and pistachios. Mix the ingredients to combine, and add the chocolate mixture to the bowl. Mix once more, then pour the mixture into the brownie tin.

4.Press the mixture with the back of a spoon to ensure it creates a flat, even layer. Refrigerate it for 2 hours, before cutting it into squares, about 4-inches in length and width.

Nutrition

130 Calories

10g Carbohydrates

1.1g Protein

40. Black Bean Balls

Preparation Time: 20 minutes

Cooking Time: 0 minute

Servings: 3

Ingredients

- 420g can black beans

- 80g raw cacao powder

- 30g almond butter

- 15ml maple syrup

Directions

1. In a food processor, combine 420g black beans, 60g cacao powder, almond butter, and maple syrup.

2Process until the mixture is well combined.

3Shape the mixture into 12 balls.

4Roll the balls through remaining cacao powder.

5Place the balls in a refrigerator for 10 minutes.

6. Serve.

Nutrition   245 Calories

17g fiber

13.1g Protein

41. Chia Soy Pudding

Preparation Time: 5 minutes

Cooking Time: 0 minute

Servings: 2

Ingredients

- 45g almond butter
- 15ml maple syrup
- ¼ teaspoon vanilla paste
- 235ml soymilk
- 45g chia seeds
- 1 small banana, sliced
- 10g crushed almonds

Direction

1Combine almond butter, maple syrup, vanilla, and soymilk in a jar.

2Stir in chia seeds.

3Cover and refrigerate 3 hours.

4After 3 hours, open the jar.

5Top the chia pudding with banana and crushed almonds.

6Serve.

Nutrition   298 Calories 10g fiber 10g Protein

42. Blueberry Ice Cream

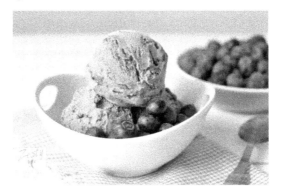

Preparation Time: 10 minutes

Cooking Time: 0 minute

Servings: 4

Ingredients

- 140g raw cashews
- 125g silken tofu
- 230g fresh blueberries
- 5g lemon zest
- 100ml maple syrup
- 100ml coconut oil
- 15g almond butter

Directions

1Rinse and drain cashews.

2Place the cashews, blueberries, pale syrup, coconut oil, and almond butter in a food processor.

3Process until smooth.

4Transfer the mixture into the freezer-friendly container.

5Seal with plastic foil and freeze for 4 hours.

6Remove the ice cream from the fridge 15 minutes before serving.

Nutrition

544 Calories

2.6g fiber

8.1g Protein

43. Chickpea Choco Slices

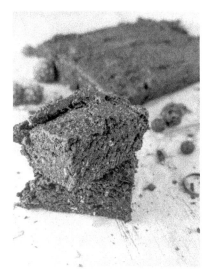

Preparation Time: 10 minutes

Cooking Time: 50 minutes

Servings: 2

Ingredients

- 400g can chickpeas
- 250g almond butter
- 70ml maple syrup
- 15ml vanilla paste
- 1 pinch salt
- 2g baking powder
- 2g baking soda
- 40g vegan chocolate chips

Directions

1Preheat oven to 180C/350F.

2Grease large baking pan with coconut oil.

3Combine chickpeas, almond butter, maple syrup, vanilla, salt, baking powder, and baking soda in a food blender.

4Blend until smooth. Stir in half the chocolate chips-

5Arrange batter into the prepared baking pan.

6Sprinkle with reserved chocolate chips.

7Bake for 45-50 minutes.

8Set aside on wire rack for 20 minutes. slice and serve.

Nutrition

426 Calories

4.9g fiber

10g Protein

CHAPTER 5:

Desserts

44. Bananas Foster

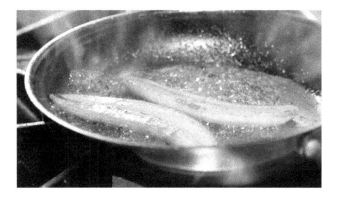

Preparation Time: 5 minutes

Cooking Time: 5 minutes

Servings: 4

Ingredients

- 2/3 cup dark brown sugar
- 1/2 teaspoons vanilla extract
- 1/2 teaspoon of ground cinnamon
- bananas, peeled and cut lengthwise and broad
- 1/4 cup chopped nuts, butter

Direction

1. Melt the butter in a deep-frying pan over medium heat. Stir in sugar, 3 ½ tbsp. of rum, vanilla, and cinnamon.

2. When the mixture starts to bubble, place the bananas and nuts in the pan. Bake until the bananas are hot, 1 to 2 minutes. Serve immediately with vanilla ice cream.

Nutrition: 534 calories 23.8g fat 4.6g protein

45. Rhubarb Strawberry Crunch

Preparation Time: 15 minutes

Cooking Time: 45 minutes

Servings: 18

Ingredients

- 3 tablespoons all-purpose flour
- 3 cups of fresh strawberries, sliced
- 3 cups of rhubarb, cut into cubes
- 1/2 cup flour
- 1 cup butter

Direction

1. Preheat the oven to 190 ° C.
2. Combine 1 cup of white sugar, 3 tablespoons flour, strawberries and rhubarb in a large bowl. Place the mixture in a 9 x 13-inch baking dish.
3. Mix 1 1/2 cups of flour, 1 cup of brown sugar, butter, and oats until a crumbly texture is obtained. You may want to use a blender for this. Crumble the mixture of rhubarb and strawberry.
4. Bake in the preheated oven for 45 minutes or until crispy and light brown.

Nutrition: 253 calories 10.8g fat 2.3g protein

46. Caramel Popcorn

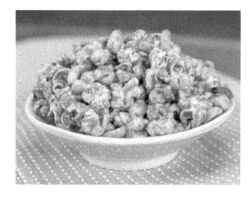

Preparation Time: 30 minutes

Cooking Time: 1 hour

Servings: 20

Ingredients

- 2 cups brown sugar
- 1/2 cup of corn syrup
- 1/2 teaspoon baking powder
- teaspoon vanilla extract
- 5 cups of popcorn

Direction

1. Preheat the oven to 95° C (250° F). Put the popcorn in a large bowl.

2. Melt 1 cup of butter in a medium-sized pan over medium heat. Stir in brown sugar, 1 tsp. of salt, and corn syrup. Bring to a boil, constantly stirring

— Cook without stirring for 4 minutes. Then remove from heat and stir in the soda and vanilla. Pour in a thin layer on the popcorn and stir well.

3. Place in two large shallow baking tins and bake in the preheated oven, stirring every 15 minutes for an hour. Remove from the oven and let cool completely before breaking into pieces.

Nutrition: 14g fat 253 calories 32.8g carbohydrates

47. Chocolate, Almond, and Cherry Clusters

Preparation Time: 15 minutes

Cooking Time: 3 minutes Serving: 5

Ingredients:

- 1 cup dark chocolate (60% cocoa or higher), chopped
- 1 tablespoon coconut oil
- ½ cup dried cherries
- 1 cup roasted salted almonds

Direction

1. Line a baking sheet with parchment paper.
2. Melt the chocolate and coconut oil in a saucepan for 3 minutes. Stir constantly.
3. Turn off the heat and mix in the cherries and almonds.
4. Drop the mixture on the baking sheet with a spoon. Place the sheet in the refrigerator and chill for at least 1 hour or until firm.
5. Serve chilled.

Nutrition: 197 calories 13.2g fat 4.1g protein

48. Chocolate and Avocado Mousse

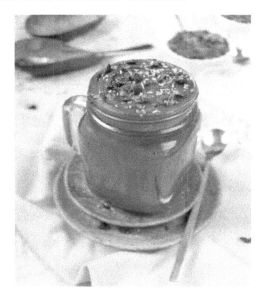

Preparation Time: 40 minutes

Cooking Time: 5 minutes

Serving: 5

Ingredients:

- 8 ounces (227 g) dark chocolate (60% cocoa or higher), chopped
- ¼ cup unsweetened coconut milk
- 2 tablespoons coconut oil
- 2 ripe avocados, deseeded

Direction:

1. Put the chocolate in a saucepan. Pour in the coconut milk and add the coconut oil.

2. Cook for 3 minutes or until the chocolate and coconut oil melt. Stir constantly.

3. Put the avocado in a food processor and melted chocolate. Pulse to combine until smooth.

4. Pour the mixture in a serving bowl, then sprinkle with salt. Refrigerate to chill for 30 minutes and serve.

Nutrition: 654 calories 46.8g fat 7.2g protein

49. French Lover's Coconut Macaroons

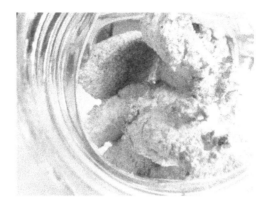

Preparation Time: 15 minutes

Cooking Time: 25 minutes

Serving: 6

Ingredients:

- 1/3 cup agave nectar

- ½ cup coconut cream

- 1 cup shredded coconut

- ½ tsp. salt

- 1/3 cup chocolate chips

Directions:

1. Begin by preheating your oven to 300 degrees Fahrenheit.

2. Next, mix together the coconut cream, the agave, and the salt. Next, fold in the chocolate chips and the coconut. Stir well, and create cookie balls. Place

the balls on a baking sheet, and bake the cookies for twenty-five minutes. Enjoy.

Nutrition

118 Calories

6g Fat

9g Protein

50. Elementary Party Vegan Oatmeal Raisin Cookies

Preparation Time: 15 minutes

Cooking Time: 35 minutes

 Serving: 12

Ingredients:

- 1 cup whole wheat flour
- ½ tsp. salt
- ½ tsp. baking soda
- 1 tsp. cinnamon
- ½ cup brown sugar
- 2 tbsp. maple syrup
- ½ cup sugar
- 1/3 cup applesauce
- ½ tsp. vanilla
- 1/3 cup olive oil
- ½ cup raisins
- 1 ¾ cup oats

Directions:

1. Begin by preheating the oven to 350 degrees Fahrenheit.

2. Next, mix together all the dry ingredients. Place this mixture to the side.

3. Next, mix together all the wet ingredients in a large mixing bowl. Add the dry ingredients to the wet ingredients slowly, stirring as you go. Add the oats next, stirring well. Lastly, add the raisins.

4. Allow the batter to chill in the refrigerator for twenty minutes. Afterwards, drop the cookies onto a baking sheet and bake them for thirteen minutes. Enjoy after cooling.

Nutrition

114 Calories

6g Fat

10g Protein

Conclusion

We hope that this book guides you to that exceptional balance between health and dieting that you have been aiming for. You are now ready to get started or continue your bodybuilding journey, and hopefully, these recipes will assist you along the way. These will also help you reach your fitness goals!

Building muscle, burning fat, and sculpting your ideal physique is easy, especially when you go all-natural and organic; it makes things tenfold easier. When you adopt a diet like this, you will typically consume less-fortified foods with much fewer calories attached.

You do not have to live this way, and now that you have seen just how delicious and mouth-watering plant-based diet meals can be, and how easy the transition to a plant-based lifestyle can be, I hope you take the steps necessary to make the switch today. Do not be confused or disheartened by the misinformation that exists about plant-based diets. Now that you know better, you can take the steps necessary to change your life and diet.

With all these recipes here in this book and the tips given to you, I hope you find the plant-based diet easy to follow. Another is that meals are delicious, not like everyone is trying to tell you.

When making a leap from other diets to plant-based diets, anything can happen along the way. Of course, there are instances where you might fall off the wagon and turn to animal-based diets or processed foods. However, what you should understand is that it is normal to fall and regress occasionally. The transformation is not easy; therefore, forgive yourself for making mistakes here and there. Concentrate on the bigger picture of living a blissful life where you are at a lower risk of cancer, diabetes, and other ailments. More importantly, keep yourself inspired by connecting with like-minded people. Do not overlook their importance in the transition, as they are also going through the challenge you are facing. Hence, they should advise you from time to time on what to do when you feel stuck.

Going vegan shouldn't be tedious. Fortunately, nature comprises of many plant foods to enjoy.

The art of turning these foods into delicious and satisfying meals is tricky, but this cookbook helps introduce you to vegan cooking if you are a beginner.

I hope you enjoyed the straightforward recipes that you can make quickly in the comfort of your home.

I look forward to sharing more vegan recipes with you in my next project.

In the meantime, have fun while you stay healthy the vegan way.

Cheers!